# The E Ketogenic Air Fryer Cookbook

Tasty and Incredibly Healthy Ketogenic Air Fryer Recipes to Enjoy Your Diet and Lose Weight

Morgan Parry

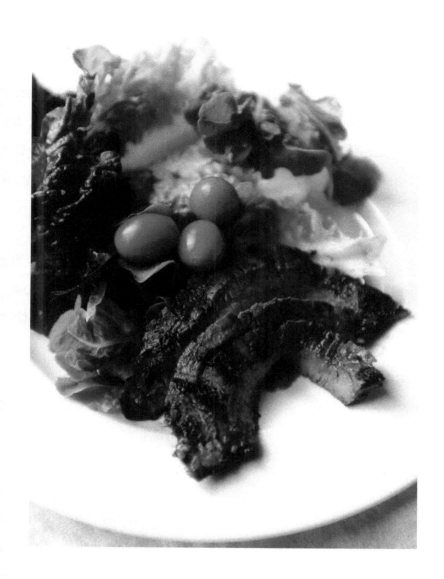

professional before attempting any techniques outlined in this book.

By reading this document, the reader agrees that under no circumstances is the author responsible for any losses, direct or indirect, which are incurred as a result of the use of information contained within this document, including, but not limited to, — errors, omissions, or inaccuracies.

# Table of Contents

# Mozzarella Chicken and Spinach

**Preparation time: 5 minutes**

**Cooking time: 24 minutes**

**Servings: 6**

## Ingredients:

- 6 chicken breasts, skinless, boneless and halved A pinch of salt and black pepper
- 2 tablespoons olive oil
- 1 pound mozzarella, sliced 2 cups baby spinach
- 1 teaspoon Italian seasoning 2 tomatoes, sliced
- 1 tablespoon basil, chopped

## Directions:

1. Make slits in each chicken breast halves, season with salt, pepper and Italian seasoning and stuff with mozzarella, spinach and tomatoes.

2. Drizzle the oil over stuffed chicken, put it in your air fryer's basket and cook at 370 degrees F for 12 minutes on each side.

3. Divide between plates and serve with basil sprinkled on top.

**Nutrition**: calories 285, fat 12, fiber 4, carbs 7, protein 15

## Pepper Turkey Bacon

**Prep time**: 10 minutes

**Cooking time**: 8 minutes

**Servings**: 2

**Ingredients**:

- 7 oz turkey bacon
- 1 teaspoon coconut oil, melted
- ½ teaspoon ground black pepper

**Directions:**

1. Slice the turkey bacon if needed and sprinkle it with ground black pepper and coconut oil. Preheat the air fryer to 400F.

2. Arrange the turkey bacon in the air fryer in one layer and cook it for 4 minutes. Then flip the bacon on another side and cook for 4 minutes more.

**Nutrition**: calories 149, fat 5.5, fiber 0.1, carbs 0.3, protein 19.3

# Duck with Olives

**Preparation time**: 5 minutes

**Cooking time**: 25 minutes

**Servings**: 2

## Ingredients:

- 2 duck legs
- 1 teaspoon cinnamon powder 1 tablespoon olive oil
- garlic clove, minced
- A pinch of salt and black pepper
- ounces black olives, pitted and sliced Juice of ½ lime
- 1 tablespoon parsley, chopped

## Directions:

1.    In a bowl, mix the duck legs with cinnamon, oil, garlic, salt and pepper, and rub well. Heat up a pan that fits the air fryer over medium-high heat, add duck legs and brown for 2-3 minutes on each side.

2.    Add the remaining ingredients to the pan, put the pan in the air fryer and cook at 400 degrees F for 10 minutes on each side. Divide between plates and serve.

**Nutrition**: calories 276, fat 12, fiber 4, carbs 6, protein 14

# Spring Chicken Mix

**Preparation time**: 10 minutes

**Cooking time**: 20 minutes

**Servings**: 4

## Ingredients:

- pounds duck breast, skinless, boneless and cubed
- ½ cup spring onions, chopped Salt and black pepper to the taste 1 tablespoon olive oil
- 2 garlic cloves, minced
- ¼ teaspoon red pepper flakes, crushed 1 tablespoons sesame seeds, toasted

## Directions:

1. Heat up a pan that fits your air fryer with the oil over medium heat, add the meat, toss and brown for 5 minutes.
2. Add the rest of the ingredients except the sesame seeds, toss, introduce in the fryer and cook at 380 degrees F for 15 minutes.
3. Add sesame seeds, toss, divide between plates and serve.

**Nutrition**: calories 264, fat 12, fiber 4, carbs 6, protein 17

# Duck and Strawberry Sauce

**Prep time**: 15 minutes

**Cooking time:** 15 minutes

**Servings**: 4

## Ingredients:

- 1-pound duck breast, skinless, boneless
- 1 tablespoon Erythritol
- 2 tablespoons water
- 1 oz strawberry
- ½ teaspoon salt
- ½ teaspoon ground paprika
- ¼ teaspoon ground cinnamon
- 1 teaspoon chili powder
- 1 teaspoon sesame oil

## Directions:

1. Rub the duck breast with salt and chili powder. Then brush it with sesame oil. Preheat the air fryer to 380F.

2.    Put the duck breast in the air fryer and cook it for 12 minutes. Meanwhile, make the sweet sauce: in the small bowl mix up Erythritol, water, ground paprika, and ground cinnamon.

3.    Mash the strawberry and add it in the Erythritol mixture. Stir it well and microwave it for 10 seconds. Then stir the sauce and microwave it for 10 seconds more.

4.    Repeat the same steps 2 times more. Then rush the duck breast with ½ part of sweet sauce and cook for 3 minutes more. Slice the cooked duck breast and sprinkle it with remaining sauce.

**Nutrition**: calories 162, fat 5.8, fiber 0.5, carbs 1.2, protein 25.1

# Chicken Satay

**Prep time**: 10 minutes

**Cooking time**: 14 minutes

**Servings**: 4

## Ingredients:

- 4 chicken wings
- 1 teaspoon olive oil
- 1 teaspoon keto tomato sauce
- 1 teaspoon dried cilantro
- ½ teaspoon salt

## Directions:

1. String the chicken wings on the wooden skewers. Then in the shallow bowl mix up olive oil, tomato sauce, dried cilantro, and salt. Spread the chicken skewers with the tomato mixture.

2. Preheat the air fryer to 390F. Arrange the chicken satay in the air fryer and cook the meal for 10 minutes. Then flip the chicken satay on another side and cook it for 4 minutes more.

**Nutrition**: calories 170, fat 11.9, fiber 0.2, carbs 5.7, protein 9.8

**Simple Paprika Duck**

**Preparation time**: 5 minutes

**Cooking time**: 25 minutes

**Servings**: 4

**Ingredients**:

• 1 pound duck breasts, skinless, boneless and cubed Salt and black pepper to the taste
• 1 tablespoon olive oil
• ½ teaspoon sweet paprika
• ¼ cup chicken stock
• 1 teaspoon thyme, chopped

**Directions**:

1. Heat up a pan that fits your air fryer with the oil over medium heat, add the duck pieces, and brown them for 5 minutes.
2. Add the rest of the ingredients, toss, put the pan in the machine and cook at 380 degrees F for 20 minutes. Divide between plates and serve.

**Nutrition**: calories 264, fat 14, fiber 4, carbs 6, protein 18

## Chicken Wings and Vinegar Sauce

**Prep time**: 10 minutes

**Cooking time**: 12 minutes

**Servings**: 4

**Ingredients**:

- 4 chicken wings
- 1 teaspoon Erythritol
- 1 teaspoon water
- 1 teaspoon apple cider vinegar
- 1 teaspoon salt
- ¼ teaspoon ground paprika
- ½ teaspoon dried oregano
- Cooking spray

**Directions**:

1.    Sprinkle the chicken wings with salt and dried oregano. Then preheat the air fryer to 400F. Place the chicken wings in the air fryer basket and cook them for 8 minutes.

2.    Flip the chicken wings on another side after 4 minutes of cooking. Meanwhile, mix up Erythritol, water,

apple cider vinegar, and ground paprika in the saucepan and bring the liquid to boil.

3.     Stir the liquid well and cook it until Erythritol is dissolved. After this, generously brush the chicken wings with sweet Erythritol liquid and cook them in the air fryer at 400F for 4 minutes more.

**Nutrition**: calories 100, fat 6.7, fiber 0.2, carbs 0.3, protein 9.2

# Celery Chicken Mix

**Prep time**: 15 minutes

**Cooking time**: 9 minutes

**Servings**: 4

## Ingredients:

- 1 teaspoon fennel seeds
- ½ teaspoon ground celery
- ½ teaspoon salt
- 1 tablespoon olive oil
- 12 oz chicken fillet

## Directions:

1. Cut the chicken fillets on 4 chicken chops. In the shallow bowl mix up fennel seeds and olive oil. Rub the chicken chops with salt and ground celery.

2. Preheat the air fryer to 365F. Brush the chicken chops with the fennel oil and place it in the air fryer basket. Cook them for 9 minutes.

**Nutrition**: calories 193, fat 9.9, fiber 0.2, carbs 0.3, protein 24.7

# Vanilla and Peppercorn Duck

**Preparation time**: 5 minutes

**Cooking time**: 30 minutes

**Servings**: 4

## Ingredients:

- 4 duck legs, skin on Juice of ½ lemon
- 1 teaspoon cinnamon powder 1 teaspoon vanilla extract
- 10 peppercorns, crushed
- 1 tablespoon balsamic vinegar 1 tablespoon olive oil
- A pinch of salt and black pepper

## Directions:

1. Heat up a pan with the oil over medium-high heat, add the duck legs and sear them for 3 minutes on each side.
2. Transfer to a pan that fits the air fryer, add the remaining ingredients, toss, put the pan in the air fryer and cook at 380 degrees F for 22 minutes. Divide duck legs and cooking juices between plates and serve.

24

**Nutrition**: calories 271, fat 13, fiber 4, carbs 6, protein 15

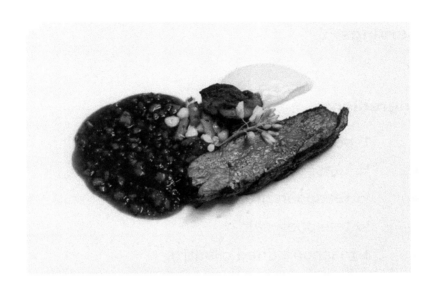

## Nutmeg Duck Meatballs

**Prep time**: 20 minutes

**Cooking time**: 10 minutes

**Servings**: 6

### Ingredients:

- 1-pound ground duck
- ½ teaspoon ground cloves
- ½ teaspoon ground nutmeg
- ½ teaspoon salt
- 1 teaspoon dried cilantro
- 2 tablespoons almond flour
- Cooking spray

### Directions:

1. In the mixing bowl mix up ground duck, ground cloves, ground nutmeg, salt, dried cilantro, and almond flour. With the help of the fingertips make the duck meatballs and sprinkle them with cooking spray.

2. Preheat the air fryer to 385F. Put the duck meatballs in the air fryer basket in one layer and cook

them for 5 minutes. Then flip the meatballs on another side and cook them for 5 minutes more.

**Nutrition**: calories 244, fat 16.3, fiber 1.7, carbs 3.4, protein 22.8

# Duck with Mushrooms and Coriander

**Preparation time**: 5 minutes

**Cooking time**: 25 minutes

**Servings**: 6

**Ingredients**:

- 6 duck breasts, boneless, skin on and scored 1 tablespoon balsamic vinegar
- 1 tablespoon coconut aminos
- A pinch of salt and black pepper 2 courgettes, sliced
- ¼ pound oyster mushrooms, sliced
- ½ bunch coriander, chopped 2 tablespoons olive oil
- garlic cloves, minced

**Directions**:

1. Heat up a pan that fits your air fryer with the oil over medium heat, add the duck breasts skin side down and sear for 5 minutes.
2. Add the rest of the ingredients, cook for 2 minutes more, transfer the pan to the air fryer and cook at 380

degrees F for 20 minutes. Divide everything between plates and serve.

**Nutrition**: calories 2764, fat 12, fiber 4, carbs 6, protein 14

# Hot Chicken Skin

**Prep time**: 10 minutes

**Cooking time**: 30 minutes

**Servings**: 4

## Ingredients:

- ½ teaspoon chili paste
- 8 oz chicken skin
- 1 teaspoon sesame oil
- ½ teaspoon chili powder
- ½ teaspoon salt

## Directions:

1.    In the shallow bowl mix up chili paste, sesame oil, chili powder, and salt. Then brush the chicken skin with chili mixture well and leave for 10 minutes to marinate.

2.    Meanwhile, preheat the air fryer to 365F. Put the marinated chicken skin in the air fryer and cook it for 20 minutes.

3.    When the time is finished, flip the chicken skin on another side and cook it for 10 minutes more or until the chicken skin is crunchy.

**Nutrition**: calories 298, fat 25.4, fiber 0.1, carbs 5.7, protein 10.9

# Duck with Peppers and Pine Nuts Sauce

**Preparation time**: 5 minutes

**Cooking time**: 25 minutes

**Servings**:  4


**Ingredients**:

- duck breast fillets, skin-on
- 1 tablespoon balsamic vinegar 4 tablespoons olive oil
- 1 red bell pepper, roasted, peeled and chopped 1/3 cup basil, chopped
- 1 tablespoon pine nuts 1 teaspoon tarragon
- 1 garlic clove, minced
- 1 tablespoon lemon juice


**Directions**:

1. Heat up a pan that fist your air fryer with half of the oil over medium heat, add the duck fillets skin side up and cook for 2-3 minutes.

2. Add the vinegar, toss and cook for 2 minutes more. In a blender, combine the rest of the oil with the remaining ingredients and pulse well. Pour this over the

duck, put the pan in the fryer and cook at 370 degrees F for 16 minutes.

3.     Divide everything between plates and serve.


**Nutrition**: calories 270, fat 14, fiber 3, carbs 6, protein 16

## Coconut Crusted Chicken

**Prep time**: 15 minutes

**Cooking time**: 9 minutes

**Servings**: 5

**Ingredients**:

- 15 oz chicken fillet
- 5 eggs, beaten
- 1 teaspoon salt
- ½ cup coconut flour
- 1 teaspoon dried oregano
- Cooking spray

**Directions**:

1.    Cut the chicken fillet on 5 chops and beat them gently with the help of the kitchen hammer. After this, sprinkle the chicken chops with dried oregano and salt.

2.    Dip every chicken chop in the beaten eggs and coat in the coconut flour. Preheat the air fryer to 360F.

3.    Place the chicken in the air fryer in one layer and cook for 5 minutes. Then flip them on another side and

cook for 4 minutes more or until the schnitzels are light brown.

**Nutrition**: calories 287, fat 12.7, fiber 4.9, carbs 7.7, protein 32.6

# Paprika Duck and Eggplant Mix

**Preparation time**: 5 minutes

**Cooking time**: 25 minutes

**Servings**: 4

## Ingredients:

•     1 pound duck breasts, skinless, boneless and cubed 2 eggplants, cubed

•     A pinch of salt and black pepper 2 tablespoons olive oil

•     1 tablespoon sweet paprika

•     ½ cup keto tomato sauce

## Directions:

1.     Heat up a pan that fits your air fryer with the oil over medium heat, add the duck pieces and brown for 5 minutes.

2.     Add the rest of the ingredients, toss, introduce the pan in the fryer and cook at 370 degrees F for 20 minutes. Divide between plates and serve.

**Nutrition**: calories 285, fat 14, fiber 4, carbs 6, protein 16

**Za'atar Chives Chicken**

**Prep time**: 10 minutes

**Cooking time**: 18 minutes

**Servings**: 4

**Ingredients**:

- 1-pound chicken drumsticks, bone-in
- 1 tablespoon zaatar
- 1 teaspoon garlic powder
- ½ teaspoon lemon zest, grated
- 1 teaspoon chives, chopped
- 1 tablespoon avocado oil

**Directions**:

1. In the mixing bowl mix up zaatar, garlic powder, lemon zest, chives, and avocado oil. Then rub the chicken drumsticks with the zaatar mixture.

2. Preheat the air fryer to 375F. Put the chicken drumsticks in the air fryer basket and cook for 15 minutes. Then flip the drumsticks on another side and cook them for 3 minutes more.

**Nutrition**: calories 201, fat 7.1, fiber 0.3, carbs 0.8, protein 31.4

## Curry Duck Mix

**Preparation time**: 5 minutes

**Cooking time**: 25 minutes

**Servings**: 4

**Ingredients**:

- 15 ounces duck breasts, skinless, boneless and cubed 1 tablespoon olive oil
- 2 shallots, chopped
- Salt and black pepper to the taste 5 ounces heavy cream
- teaspoon curry powder
- ½ bunch coriander, chopped

**Directions**:

1. Heat up a pan that fits your air fryer with the oil over medium heat, add the duck, toss and brown for 5 minutes.
2. Add the rest of the ingredients, toss, introduce the pan in the air fryer and cook at 370 degrees F for 20 minutes. Divide the mix into bowls and serve.

**Nutrition**: calories 274, fat 14, fiber 4, carbs 7, protein 16

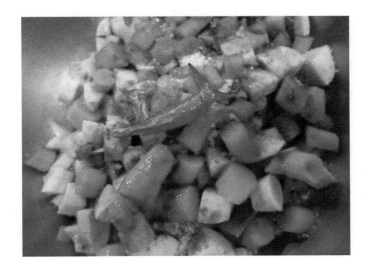

## Yogurt Chicken Thighs

**Prep time**: 25 minutes

**Cooking time**: 20 minutes

**Servings**: 4

### Ingredients:

- 4 chicken thighs, skinless, boneless
- 2 tablespoons plain yogurt
- 1 teaspoon cayenne pepper
- 1 teaspoon dried cilantro
- ½ teaspoon ground cloves
- 1 tablespoon apple cider vinegar
- 1 teaspoon olive oil

### Directions:

1. Make the marinade: in the mixing bowl mix up plain yogurt, cayenne pepper, dried cilantro, ground cloves, and apple cider vinegar. Then put the chicken thighs in the marinade and mix up well.

2. Marinate the chicken for 20 minutes in the fridge. Then preheat the air fryer to 380F. Sprinkle the chicken

thighs with olive oil and place in the air fryer. Cook them for 20 minutes.

**Nutrition**: calories 296, fat 12.2, fiber 0.2, carbs 1, protein 42.8

# Duck and Asparagus Mix

**Preparation time**: 5 minutes

**Cooking time**: 25 minutes

**Servings**:  4

**Ingredients**:

- duck breast fillets, boneless
- ½ cup keto tomato sauce A drizzle of olive oil
- Salt and black pepper to the taste 1 cup red bell pepper, chopped
- ½ pound asparagus, trimmed and halved
- ½ cup cheddar cheese, grated

**Directions**:

1.    Heat up a pan that fits your air fryer with the oil over medium heat, add the duck fillets and brown for 5 minutes.

2.    Add the rest of the ingredients except the cheese, toss, put the pan in the air fryer and cook at 370 degrees F for 20 minutes.

3.    Sprinkle the cheese on top, divide the mix between plates and serve.

**Nutrition**: calories 263, fat 12, fiber 4, carbs 6, protein 14

# Rosemary Partridge

**Prep time**: 15 minutes

**Cooking time**: 14 minutes

**Servings**: 4

## Ingredients:

- 10 oz partridges
- 1 teaspoon dried rosemary
- 1 tablespoon butter, melted
- 1 teaspoon salt

## Directions:

1.  Cut the partridges into the halves and sprinkle with dried rosemary and salt. Then brush them with melted butter.
2.  Preheat the air fryer to 385F. Put the partridge halves in the air fryer and cook them for 8 minutes.
3.  Then flip the poultry on another side and cook for 6 minutes more.

**Nutrition**: calories 175, fat 7.8, fiber 0.1, carbs 0.2, protein 25.2

# Duck and Lettuce Salad

**Preparation time**: 5 minutes

**Cooking time**: 20 minutes

**Servings**: 4

## Ingredients:

- 2 duck breasts, boneless and skin on 1 teaspoon coconut oil, melted
- A pinch of salt and black pepper 2 shallots, sliced
- 12 cherry tomatoes, halved
- 1 tablespoon balsamic vinegar 3 cups lettuce leaves, torn
- 12 mint leaves, torn

## For the dressing:

- 1 tablespoon lemon juice
- ½ tablespoon balsamic vinegar 2 and ½ tablespoons olive oil
- ½ teaspoon mustard

**Directions**:

1.     Heat up a pan that fits your air fryer with the coconut oil over medium heat, add the duck breasts skin side down and cook for 3 minutes. Add salt, pepper, shallots, tomatoes and 1 tablespoon balsamic vinegar, toss, put the pan in the fryer and cook at 370 degrees F for 17 minutes.

2.     Cool this mix down, thinly slice the duck breast and put it along with the tomatoes and shallots in a bowl. Add mint and salad leaves and toss. In a separate bowl, mix ½ tablespoon vinegar with lemon juice, oil and mustard and whisk well. Pour this over the duck salad, toss and serve.

**Nutrition**: calories 241, fat 10, fiber 2, carbs 5, protein 15

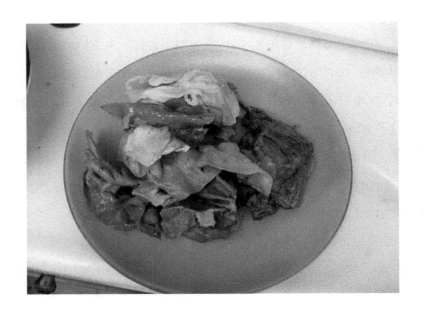

# Ginger Partridges

**Prep time**: 15 minutes

**Cooking time**: 20 minutes

**Servings**: 6

## Ingredients:

- 18 oz partridges, trimmed
- 3 oz bacon, sliced
- 1 teaspoon minced ginger
- 1 tablespoon avocado oil
- ½ teaspoon garlic powder
- 1 teaspoon salt
- ½ teaspoon smoked paprika

## Directions:

1.     Rub the partridges with minced ginger and sprinkle with garlic powder, salt, and smoked paprika.

2.     Then wrap the poultry in the sliced bacon and sprinkle with avocado oil. Preheat the air fryer to 375F. Place the wrapped partridges in the air fryer basket and cook them for 20 minutes. Flip them on another side after 10 minutes of cooking.

**Nutrition**: calories 260, fat 12.1, fiber 0.2, carbs 0.8, protein 35.6

# Balsamic Duck and Cranberry Sauce

**Preparation time**: 5 minutes

**Cooking time**: 25 minutes

**Servings**: 4

## Ingredients:

- 4 duck breasts, boneless, skin-on and scored A pinch of salt and black pepper
- 1 tablespoon olive oil
- ¼ cup balsamic vinegar
- ½ cup dried cranberries

## Directions:

1. Heat up a pan that fits your air fryer with the oil over medium-high heat, add the duck breasts skin side down and cook for 5 minutes.

2. Add the rest of the ingredients, toss, put the pan in the fryer and cook at 380 degrees F for 20 minutes. Divide between plates and serve.

**Nutrition**: calories 287, fat 12, fiber 4, carbs 6, protein
16

## Stuffed Chicken

**Prep time**: 15 minutes

**Cooking time**: 11 minutes

**Servings**: 2


**Ingredients**:

- 8 oz chicken fillet
- 3 oz Blue cheese
- ½ teaspoon salt
- ½ teaspoon thyme
- 1 teaspoon sesame oil


**Directions**:

1. Cut the fillet into halves and beat them gently with the help of the kitchen hammer. After this, make the horizontal cut in every fillet. Sprinkle the chicken with salt and thyme.

2. Then fill it with Blue cheese and secure the cut with the help of the toothpick. Sprinkle the stuffed chicken fillets with sesame oil.

3. Preheat the air fryer to 385F. Put the chicken fillets in the air fryer and cook them for 7 minutes. Then

carefully flip the chicken fillets on another side and cook for 4 minutes more.


**Nutrition**: calories 386, fat 22.9, fiber 0.1, carbs 1.2, protein 41.9

**Parsley Duck**

**Preparation time**: 10 minutes

**Cooking time**: 25 minutes

**Servings**: 4

**Ingredients**:

- 4 duck breast fillets, boneless, skin-on and scored 2 tablespoons olive oil
- 2 tablespoons parsley, chopped Salt and black pepper to the taste 1 cup chicken stock
- 1 teaspoon balsamic vinegar

**Directions**:

1. Heat up a pan that fits your air fryer with the oil over medium heat, add the duck breasts skin side down and sear for 5 minutes.
2. Add the rest of the ingredients, toss, put the pan in the fryer and cook at 380 degrees F for 20 minutes. Divide everything between plates and serve

**Nutrition**: calories 274, fat 14, fiber 4, carbs 6, protein 16

# Fried Herbed Chicken Wings

**Prep time**: 10 minutes

**Cooking time**: 11 minutes

**Servings**: 4

## Ingredients:

- 1 tablespoon Emperor herbs chicken spices
- 8 chicken wings
- Cooking spray

## Directions:

1. Generously sprinkle the chicken wings with Emperor herbs chicken spices and place in the preheated to 400F air fryer. Cook the chicken wings for 6 minutes from each side.

**Nutrition**: calories 220, fat 14.3, fiber 0.6, carbs 3.9, protein 17.7

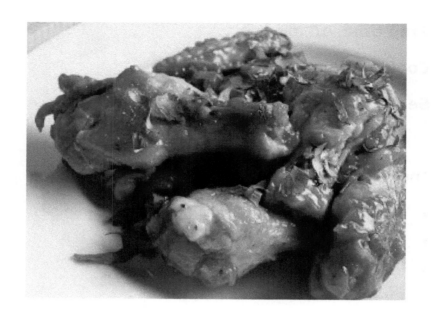

# Duck and Coconut Milk Mix

**Preparation time**: 5 minutes

**Cooking time**: 25 minutes

**Servings**: 4

## Ingredients:

- garlic cloves, minced
- duck breasts, boneless, skin-on and scored 2 tablespoons olive oil
- ¼ teaspoon coriander, ground 14 ounces coconut milk
- Salt and black pepper to the taste 1 cup basil, chopped

## Directions:

1. Heat up a pan that fits your air fryer with the oil over medium heat, add the duck breasts, skin side down and sear for 5 minutes.
2. Add the rest of the ingredients, toss, put the pan in the fryer and cook at 380 degrees F for 20 minutes. Divide between plates and serve.

**Nutrition**: calories 274, fat 13, fiber 3, carbs 5, protein 16

# Lemongrass Hens

**Prep time**: 20 minutes

**Cooking time**: 65 minutes

**Cooking time**: 4

**Ingredients**:

- 14 oz hen (chicken)
- 1 teaspoon lemongrass
- 1 teaspoon ground coriander
- 1 oz celery stalk, chopped
- 1 teaspoon dried cilantro
- 3 spring onions, diced
- 2 tablespoons avocado oil
- 2 tablespoons lime juice
- ½ teaspoon lemon zest, grated
- 1 teaspoon salt
- 1 tablespoon apple cider vinegar
- 1 teaspoon chili powder
- ½ teaspoon ground black pepper

**Directions**:

1.	In the mixing bowl mix up lemongrass, ground coriander, dried cilantro, lime juice, lemon zest, salt, apple cider vinegar, and ground black pepper.

2.	Then add spring onions and celery stalk. After this, rub the hen with the spice mixture and leave for 10 minutes to marinate.

3.	Meanwhile, preheat the air fryer to 375F. Put the hen in the air fryer and cook it for 55 minutes. Then flip it on another side and cook for 10 minutes more.

**Nutrition**: calories 177, fat 4.1, fiber 1.41, carbs 4.4, protein 29.3

# Paprika Chicken Breasts

**Preparation time: 5 minutes**

**Cooking time: 20 minutes**

**Servings: 4**

**Ingredients:**

- 4 chicken breasts, skinless and boneless 1 teaspoon chili powder
- A pinch of salt and black pepper A drizzle of olive oil
- 1 teaspoon smoked paprika 1 teaspoon garlic powder
- 1 tablespoon parsley, chopped

**Directions:**

1. Season chicken with salt and pepper, and rub it with the oil and all the other ingredients except the parsley.
2. Put the chicken breasts in your air fryer's basket and cook at 350 degrees F for 10 minutes on each side.
3. Divide between plates, sprinkle the parsley on top and serve.

**Nutrition**: calories 222, fat 11, fiber 4, carbs 6, protein 12

# Provolone Meatballs

**Prep time**: 10 minutes

**Cooking time**: 12 minutes

**Servings**: 6

**Ingredients**:

- 12 oz ground chicken
- ½ cup coconut flour
- 2 egg whites, whisked
- 1 teaspoon ground black pepper
- 1 egg yolk
- 1 teaspoon salt
- 4 oz Provolone cheese, grated
- 1 teaspoon ground oregano
- ½ teaspoon chili powder
- 1 tablespoon avocado oil

**Directions**:

1.    In the mixing bowl mix up ground chicken, ground black pepper, egg yolk, salt, Provolone cheese, ground oregano, and chili powder. Stir the mixture until homogenous and make the small meatballs.

2.   Dip the meatballs in the whisked egg whites and coat in the coconut flour. Preheat the air fryer to 370F. Put the chicken meatballs in the air fryer basket and cook them for 6 minutes from both sides.

**Nutrition**: calories 234, fat 11.7, fiber 3.7, carbs 6.6, protein 24.3

# Thyme and Okra Chicken Thighs

**Preparation time: 5 minutes**

**Cooking time: 30 minutes**

**Servings: 4**

## Ingredients:

• 4 chicken thighs, bone-in and skinless A pinch of salt and black pepper

• 1 cup okra

• ½ cup butter, melted Zest of 1 lemon, grated 4 garlic cloves, minced

• tablespoon thyme, chopped 1 tablespoon parsley, chopped

## Directions:

1. Heat up a pan that fits your air fryer with half of the butter over medium heat, add the chicken thighs and brown them for 2-3 minutes on each side. Add the rest of the butter, the okra and all the remaining ingredients, toss, put the pan in the air fryer and cook at 370 degrees F for 20 minutes.

2. Divide between plates and serve.

**Nutrition**: calories 270, fat 12, fiber 4, carbs 6, protein 14

# Lemon and Chili Chicken Drumsticks

**Prep time**: 10 minutes

**Cooking time**: 20 minutes

**Servings**: 6

**Ingredients**:

- 6 chicken drumsticks
- 1 teaspoon dried oregano
- 1 tablespoon lemon juice
- ½ teaspoon lemon zest, grated
- 1 teaspoon ground cumin
- ½ teaspoon chili flakes
- 1 teaspoon garlic powder
- ½ teaspoon ground coriander
- 1 tablespoon avocado oil

**Directions**:

1. Rub the chicken drumsticks with dried oregano, lemon juice, lemon zest, ground cumin, chili flakes, garlic powder, and ground coriander.

2.    Then sprinkle them with avocado oil and put in the air fryer. Cook the chicken drumsticks for 20 minutes at 375F.

**Nutrition**: calories 85, fat 3.1, fiber 0.3, carbs 0.9, protein 12.9

# Garlic Chicken Wings

**Preparation time: 5 minutes**

**Cooking time: 30 minutes**

**Servings: 4**

**Ingredients:**

pounds chicken wings

¼ cup olive oil Juice of 2 lemons

Zest of 1 lemon, grated

A pinch of salt and black pepper 2 garlic cloves, minced

**Directions:**

1.    In a bowl, mix the chicken wings with the rest of the ingredients and toss well.

2.    Put the chicken wings in your air fryer's basket and cook at 400 degrees F for 30 minutes, shaking halfway. Divide between plates and serve with a side salad.

**Nutrition**: calories 263, fat 14, fiber 4, carbs 6, protein 15

# Cream Cheese Chicken Mix

**Prep time**: 15 minutes

**Cooking time**: 16 minutes

**Servings**: 4

## Ingredients:

- 1-pound chicken wings
- ¼ cup cream cheese
- 1 tablespoon apple cider vinegar
- 1 teaspoon Truvia
- ½ teaspoon smoked paprika
- ½ teaspoon ground nutmeg
- 1 teaspoon avocado oil

## Directions:

1.   In the mixing bowl mix up cream cheese, Truvia, apple cider vinegar, smoked paprika, and ground nutmeg.

2.   Then add the chicken wings and coat them in the cream cheese mixture well. Leave the chicken winds in the cream cheese mixture for 10-15 minutes to marinate.

3.    Meanwhile, preheat the air fryer to 380F. Put the chicken wings in the air fryer and cook them for 8 minutes.

4.    Then flip the chicken wings on another and brush with cream cheese marinade. Cook the chicken wings for 8 minutes more.


**Nutrition**: calories 271, fat 13.7, fiber 0.2, carbs 1.2, protein 34

# Buttery Chicken Wings

**Preparation time: 5 minutes**

**Cooking time: 30 minutes**

**Servings: 4**

## Ingredients:

- pounds chicken wings
- Salt and black pepper to the taste 3 garlic cloves, minced
- tablespoons butter, melted
- ½ cup heavy cream
- ½ teaspoon basil, dried
- ½ teaspoon oregano, dried
- ¼ cup parmesan, grated

## Directions:

1. In a baking dish that fits your air fryer, mix the chicken wings with all the ingredients except the parmesan and toss.
2. Put the dish to your air fryer and cook at 380 degrees F for 30 minutes. Sprinkle the cheese on top,

leave the mix aside for 10 minutes, divide between plates and serve.


**Nutrition**: calories 270, fat 12, fiber 3, carbs 6, protein 17

# Parmesan and Dill Chicken

**Prep time**: 15 minutes

**Cooking time**: 20 minutes

**Servings**: 6


## Ingredients:

- 18 oz chicken breast, skinless, boneless
- 5 oz pork rinds
- 3 oz Parmesan, grated
- 3 eggs, beaten
- 1 teaspoon chili flakes
- 1 teaspoon ground paprika
- 2 tablespoons avocado oil
- 1 teaspoon Erythritol
- ¼ teaspoon onion powder
- 1 teaspoon cayenne pepper
- 1 chili pepper, minced
- ½ teaspoon dried dill

**Directions**:

1.     In the shallow bowl mix up chili flakes, ground paprika, Erythritol. Onion powder, and cayenne pepper. Add dried dill and stir the mixture gently.

2.     Then rub the chicken breast in the spice mixture. Then rub the chicken with minced chili pepper. Dip the chicken breast in the beaten eggs. After this, coat it in the Parmesan and dip in the eggs again.

3.     Then coat the chicken in the pork rinds and sprinkle with avocado oil. Preheat the air fryer to 380F. Put the chicken breast in the air fryer and cook it for 16 minutes.

4.     Then flip the chicken breast on another side and cook it for 4 minutes more.


**Nutrition**: calories 318, fat 16.5, fiber 0.5, carbs 1.5, protein 40.7

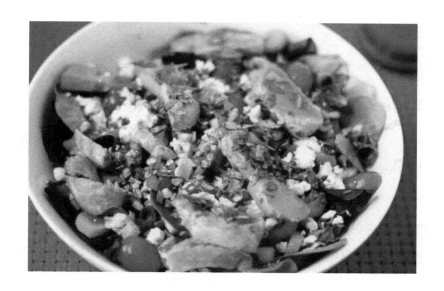

**Ginger and Coconut Chicken**

**Preparation time:** 5 minutes

**Cooking time:** 20 minutes

**Servings:** 4

**Ingredients**:

•      chicken breasts, skinless, boneless and halved 4 tablespoons coconut aminos

•      1 teaspoon olive oil 2 tablespoons stevia

•      Salt and black pepper to the taste

•      ¼ cup chicken stock

•      1 tablespoon ginger, grated

**Directions**:

1.      In a pan that fits the air fryer, combine the chicken with the ginger and all the ingredients and toss.

2.      Put the pan in your air fryer and cook at 4380 degrees F for 20, shaking the fryer halfway. Divide between plates and serve with a side salad.

**Nutrition**: calories 256, fat 12, fiber 4, carbs 6, protein 14

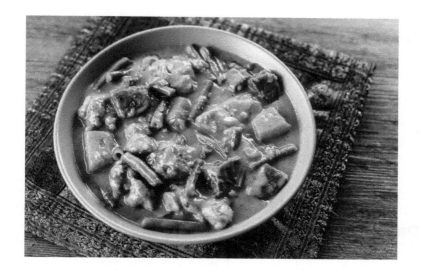

# Tomato Chicken Mix

**Prep time**: 10 minutes

**Cooking time**: 18 minutes

**Servings**: 4

**Ingredients**:

- 1-pound chicken breast, skinless, boneless
- 1 tablespoon keto tomato sauce
- 1 teaspoon avocado oil
- ½ teaspoon garlic powder

**Directions**:

1.   In the small bowl mix up tomato sauce, avocado oil, and garlic powder. Then brush the chicken breast with the tomato sauce mixture well. Preheat the air fryer to 385F.

2.   Place the chicken breast in the air fryer and cook it for 15 minutes. Then flip it on another side and cook for 3 minutes more. Slice the cooked chicken breast into Servings.

**Nutrition**: calories 139, fat 3, fiber 0.2, carbs 2, protein 24.2

# Chicken with Asparagus and Zucchini

**Preparation time:** 15 minutes

**Cooking time:** 25 minutes

**Servings:** 4

**Ingredients:**

- pound chicken thighs, boneless and skinless Juice of 1 lemon
- tablespoons olive oil 3 garlic cloves, minced
- 1 teaspoon oregano, dried
- ½ pound asparagus, trimmed and halved A pinch of salt and black pepper
- 1 zucchinis, halved lengthwise and sliced into half-moons

**Directions:**

1.    In a bowl, mix the chicken with all the ingredients except the asparagus and the zucchinis, toss and leave aside for 15 minutes.

2.    Add the zucchinis and the asparagus, toss, put everything into a pan that fits the air fryer, and cook at 380 degrees F for 25 minutes. Divide everything between plates and serve.

**Nutrition**: calories 280, fat 11, fiber 4, carbs 6, protein 17

# Coconut Chicken

**Prep time**: 15 minutes

**Cooking time**: 12 minutes

**Servings**: 4

## Ingredients:

- 12 oz chicken fillet (3 oz each fillet)
- 4 teaspoons coconut flakes
- 1 egg white, whisked
- 1 teaspoon salt
- ½ teaspoon ground black pepper
- Cooking spray

## Directions:

1.    Beat the chicken fillets with the kitchen hammer and sprinkle with salt and ground black pepper. Then dip every chicken chop in the whisked egg white and coat in the coconut flakes. Preheat the air fryer to 360F.

2.    Put the chicken chops in the air fryer and spray with cooking spray. Cook the chicken chop for 7 minutes.

3.    Then flip them on another side and cook for 5 minutes. The cooked chicken chops should have a golden brown color.

**Nutrition**: calories 172, fat 6.9, fiber 0.2, carbs 0.5, protein 25.6

# Chicken and Olives Mix

**Preparation time:** 10 minutes

**Cooking time:** 30 minutes

**Servings:** 4

**Ingredients**:

- 8 chicken thighs, boneless and skinless A pinch of salt and black pepper
- 2 tablespoons olive oil
- 1 teaspoon oregano, dried
- ½ teaspoon garlic powder
- 1 cup pepperoncini, drained and sliced
- ½ cup black olives, pitted and sliced
- ½ cup kalamata olives, pitted and sliced
- ¼ cup parmesan, grated

Directions:

1. Heat up a pan that fits the air fryer with the oil over medium-high heat, add the chicken and brown for 2 minutes on each side.

2. Add salt, pepper, and all the other ingredients except the parmesan and toss. Put the pan in the air

fryer, sprinkle the parmesan on top and cook at 370 degrees F for 25 minutes. Divide the chicken mix between plates and serve.

**Nutrition**: calories 270, fat 14, fiber 4, carbs 6, protein 18

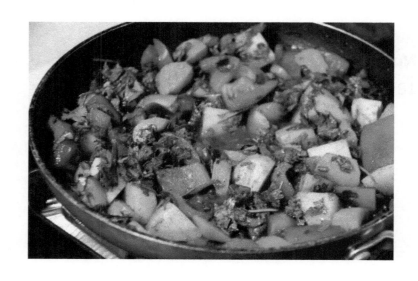

## Chicken and Ghee Mix

**Prep time**: 15 minutes

**Cooking time**: 30 minutes

**Servings**: 4

**Ingredients**:

- 12 oz chicken legs
- 1 teaspoon yeast
- 1 teaspoon chili flakes
- ½ teaspoon ground cumin
- ½ teaspoon garlic powder
- 1 teaspoon ground turmeric
- ½ teaspoon ground paprika
- 1 teaspoon Splenda
- ¼ cup coconut flour
- 1 tablespoon ghee, melted

Directions:

1. In the mixing bowl mix up yeast, chili flakes, ground cumin, garlic powder, ground turmeric, ground paprika, Splenda, and coconut flour.

2.　　Then brush every chicken leg with ghee and coat well in the coconut flour mixture. Preheat the air fryer to 380F. Place the chicken legs in the air fryer in one layer. Cook them for 15 minutes.

3.　　Then flip the chicken legs on another side and cook them for 15 minutes more.

**Nutrition**: calories 238, fat 10.9, fiber 3.5, carbs 6.8, protein 26.7

**Pesto Chicken**

**Preparation time: 10 minutes**

**Cooking time: 25 minutes**

**Servings: 4**

**Ingredients**:

- cup basil pesto
- tablespoons olive oil
- A pinch of salt and black pepper 1 and ½ pounds chicken wings

**Directions**:

1. In a bowl, mix the chicken wings with all the ingredients and toss well. Put the meat in the air fryer's basket and cook at 380 degrees F for 25 minutes. Divide between plates and serve.

**Nutrition**: calories 244, fat 11, fiber 4, carbs 6, protein 17

## Hoisin Chicken

**Prep time**: 25 minutes

**Cooking time**: 22 minutes

**Servings**: 4

**Ingredients**:

- ½ teaspoon hoisin sauce
- ½ teaspoon salt
- ½ teaspoon chili powder
- ½ teaspoon ground black pepper
- ½ teaspoon ground cumin
- ¼ teaspoon xanthan gum
- 1 teaspoon apple cider vinegar
- 1 tablespoon sesame oil
- 3 tablespoons coconut cream
- ½ teaspoon minced garlic
- ½ teaspoon chili paste
- 1-pound chicken drumsticks
- 2 tablespoons almond flour

**Directions**:

1.     Rub the chicken drumsticks with salt, chili powder, ground black pepper, ground cumin, and leave for 10 minutes to marinate. Meanwhile, in the mixing bowl mix up chili paste, minced garlic, coconut cream, apple cider vinegar, xanthan gum, and almond flour.

2.     Coat the chicken drumsticks in the coconut cream mixture well, and leave to marinate for 10 minutes more. Preheat the air fryer to 375F.

3.     Put the chicken drumsticks in the air fryer and cook them for 22 minutes.

**Nutrition**: calories 279, fat 14.5, fiber 1.7, carbs 3.4, protein 32.4

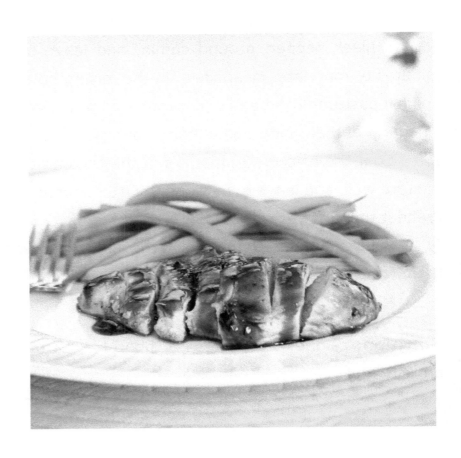

# Sun-dried Tomatoes and Chicken Mix

**Preparation time**: 5 minutes

**Cooking time:** 25 minutes

**Servings: 4**

**Ingredients**:

- 4 chicken thighs, skinless, boneless 1 tablespoon olive oil
- A pinch of salt and black pepper 1 tablespoon thyme, chopped
- 1 cup chicken stock
- 3 garlic cloves, minced
- ½ cup coconut cream
- cup sun-dried tomatoes, chopped 4 tablespoons parmesan, grated

**Directions**:

1. Heat up a pan that fits the air fryer with the oil over medium-high heat, add the chicken, salt, pepper and the garlic, and brown for 2-3 minutes on each side.

2. Add the rest of the ingredients except the parmesan, toss, put the pan in the air fryer and cook at

370 degrees F for 20 minutes. Sprinkle the parmesan on top, leave the mix aside for 5 minutes, divide everything between plates and serve.

**Nutrition**: calories 275, fat 12, fiber 4, carbs 6, protein 17

## Cauliflower Stuffed Chicken

**Prep time**: 20 minutes

**Cooking time**: 25 minutes

**Servings**: 5

**Ingredients**:

- 1 ½-pound chicken breast, skinless, boneless
- ½ cup cauliflower, shredded
- 1 jalapeno pepper, chopped
- 1 teaspoon ground nutmeg
- 1 teaspoon salt
- ¼ cup Cheddar cheese, shredded
- ½ teaspoon cayenne pepper
- 1 tablespoon cream cheese
- 1 tablespoon sesame oil
- ½ teaspoon dried thyme

**Directions**:

1.    Make the horizontal cut in the chicken breast. In the mixing bowl mix up shredded cauliflower, chopped jalapeno pepper, ground nutmeg, salt, and cayenne pepper.

2. Fill the chicken cut with the shredded cauliflower and secure the cut with toothpicks. Then rub the chicken breast with cream cheese, dried thyme, and sesame oil.

3. Preheat the air fryer to 380F. Put the chicken breast in the air fryer and cook it for 20 minutes. Then sprinkle it with Cheddar cheese and cook for 5 minutes more.

**Nutrition**: calories 266, fat 9.6, fiber 0.5, carbs 1.2, protein 41.3

# Ginger Chicken and Lemon Sauce

**Preparation time**: 5 minutes

**Cooking time**: 25 minutes

**Servings**: 4


**Ingredients**:

- tablespoons spring onions, minced 1 tablespoon ginger, grated
- 4 garlic cloves, minced
- 2 tablespoons coconut aminos 8 chicken drumsticks
- ½ cup chicken stock
- Salt and black pepper to the taste 1 teaspoon olive oil
- ¼ cup cilantro, chopped 1 tablespoon lemon juice


**Directions**:

1. Heat up a pan with the oil over medium-high heat, add the chicken drumsticks, brown them for 2 minutes on each side and transfer to a pan that fits the fryer.

2. Add all the other ingredients, toss everything, put the pan in the fryer and cook at 370 degrees F for 20

minutes. Divide the chicken and lemon sauce between plates and serve.

**Nutrition**: calories 267, fat 11, fiber 4, carbs 6, protein 16

## Dill Chicken Quesadilla

**Prep time**: 15 minutes

**Cooking time**: 10 minutes

**Servings**: 2

### Ingredients:

- 2 low carb tortillas
- 7 oz chicken breast, skinless, boneless, boiled
- 1 tablespoon cream cheese
- 1 teaspoon butter, melted
- 1 teaspoon minced garlic
- 1 teaspoon fresh dill, chopped
- ½ teaspoon salt
- 2 oz Monterey Jack cheese, shredded
- Cooking spray

### Directions:

1.    Shred the chicken breast with the help of the fork and put it in the bowl. Add cream cheese, butter, minced garlic, dill, and salt.

2.    Add shredded Monterey jack cheese and stir the shredded chicken.

3.    Then put 1 tortilla in the air fryer baking pan. Top it with the shredded chicken mixture and cover with the second corn tortilla. Cook the meal for 5 minutes at 400F.

**Nutrition**: calories 337, fat 16.7, fiber 7.1, carbs 13.1, Protein 31.6

Lightning Source UK Ltd.
Milton Keynes UK
UKHW020731210621
385887UK00005B/124